The Newly Diagnosed Kidney Disease Cookbook

Delicious Recipes to Combat Chronic Kidney Disease

MICHAEL B. HERBERT

Table of Contents

<u>Introduction</u>

Chapter 1: Overview of Kidney Disease

<u>What Is Kidney Disease?</u>

<u>Causes of Kidney Disease</u>

<u>Symptoms of Kidney Disease</u>

Chapter 2: Understanding Chronic Kidney Disease

<u>Diagnosis of Chronic Kidney Disease</u>

<u>Treatment and Management of Chronic Kidney Disease</u>

Chapter 3: Nutrition and Diet in Chronic Kidney Disease

The Basics of Nutrition and Diet in Chronic Kidney Disease

Low Sodium Diet

Low Potassium Diet

Low Phosphorous Diet

Low Protein Diet

Fluid Restriction

Chapter 4: Recipes for Chronic Kidney Disease

Breakfast Recipes

Lunch Recipes

Dinner Recipes

<u>Snack Recipes</u>

<u>Dessert Recipes</u>

Conclusion

Introduction

When my mother was diagnosed with chronic kidney disease, the first thing that came to my mind was how it would affect her diet. As a foodie, she loved exploring new recipes and trying out different cuisines. To my surprise, she was still able to enjoy her favorite dishes while following the prescribed diet. She found that with a few minor adjustments, she could still prepare delicious meals that would not only be beneficial for her health but also enjoyable to eat. This cookbook is dedicated to all those who, like my mother, have been newly diagnosed with kidney disease and are looking for recipes that are both delicious and healthy.

Kidney disease is a serious condition that affects millions of people around the world. It can be a scary diagnosis and can seem overwhelming when you first learn about it. But it doesn't have to be all doom and gloom. With the right diet, lifestyle changes, and recipes, you can still eat delicious food while managing your kidney disease.

The Newly Diagnosed Kidney Disease Cookbook is here to help you do just that. This cookbook is filled with delicious recipes to combat chronic kidney disease and help you stay healthy. Each recipe has been carefully crafted to provide nutrition while avoiding the ingredients that can be harmful to your kidneys. We've also included tips and advice on how to make the most out of your diet and make healthy decisions.

So whether you've just been diagnosed or if you're looking for a new way to manage your kidney disease, this cookbook has something for everyone. With our wide variety of recipes, you'll be able to find the perfect dish to suit your needs. So let's get cooking and make eating with kidney disease easy and delicious!

It's time to take control of your kidney disease and enjoy the food you eat with The Newly Diagnosed Kidney Disease Cookbook.

Let's get started!

Chapter 1: Overview of Kidney Disease

What Is Kidney Disease?

Kidney disease is a general term used to describe any condition that affects the normal functioning of the kidneys, including glomerulonephritis, nephrotic syndrome, and chronic kidney disease. The kidneys are vital organs that have a number of important functions in the body. They filter out waste products from the bloodstream, regulate the body's salt, potassium and acid-base balance, and produce hormones that control blood pressure and red blood cell production. When the kidneys are damaged, these functions can be impaired.

Kidney diseases can be divided into two categories: acute and chronic. Acute kidney disease is usually caused by an infection or injury, and is usually reversible with treatment. Chronic kidney disease is a progressive, long-term condition that develops over time and can be caused by a variety of factors, including diabetes, high blood pressure, and other illnesses.

Symptoms of kidney disease include swelling in the hands and feet, fatigue, difficulty concentrating, loss of appetite, and frequent urination. In advanced stages, kidney disease can lead to kidney failure, which requires dialysis or a kidney transplant to treat. Treatment of kidney disease often depends on the cause, but may include lifestyle changes, medications, and in some cases, surgery.

The best way to prevent kidney disease is to maintain a healthy lifestyle, including eating a balanced diet, exercising regularly, avoiding tobacco and excessive alcohol use, and controlling chronic conditions such as diabetes and high blood pressure. Regular screening tests can help to identify early signs of kidney disease and allow for prompt treatment. Early detection and treatment of kidney disease can help to reduce the risk of complications.

Causes of Kidney Disease

Kidney disease is a serious health condition which affects millions of people worldwide. It can be caused by a variety of factors, including genetics, lifestyle, and environmental factors. Kidney disease can lead to a number of serious health problems, including kidney failure, which can be life-threatening.

The most common causes of kidney disease include:

1. Diabetes: Diabetes is one of the most common causes of kidney disease. People with diabetes are at higher risk of developing kidney disease due to the high levels of glucose in their blood. Over time,

high levels of glucose can damage the kidneys, leading to kidney failure.

2. High Blood Pressure: High blood pressure is another major cause of kidney disease. Chronic high blood pressure can cause the arteries in the kidneys to become narrowed, reducing blood flow to the kidneys. Over time, this can lead to kidney damage and failure.

3. Infections: Infections of the urinary tract, such as bladder infections, can also cause kidney damage. The bacteria that cause these infections can enter the kidneys and cause damage to the tissue.

4. Genetics: Genetics can also play a role in the development of kidney disease. Some people are born with kidney diseases due to genetic abnormalities. Some people may also be at higher risk for developing kidney disease due to their family history.

5. Kidney Stones: Kidney stones are another common cause of kidney disease. Kidney stones form when minerals and other substances harden in the kidneys, blocking the passage of urine. This can cause pain and other symptoms, as well as kidney damage.

6. Medications: Certain medications, such as non-steroidal anti-inflammatory drugs (NSAIDs) and some antibiotics, can damage the kidneys over time. Taking these medications in excess or over a long period of time can lead to kidney damage.

7. Heavy Metal Toxicity: Heavy metals, such as lead, mercury, and cadmium, can accumulate in the body and cause kidney damage. People who are exposed to these metals through their work or lifestyle may be at higher risk for developing kidney disease.

8. Other Causes: Other causes of kidney disease include chronic dehydration, high levels of calcium in the blood, and long-term alcohol use.

In conclusion, kidney disease is a serious condition that can have serious consequences if left untreated. Identifying and addressing the underlying causes of kidney disease is the key to preventing and treating the condition.

Symptoms of Kidney Disease

The most common symptoms that may signify kidney disease include:

1. Changes in Urination: People with kidney disease may experience changes in the amount and frequency of urination. They may urinate more often and in larger amounts than usual. Alternatively, they may urinate less often and in smaller amounts than normal. Changes in the color or odor of

the urine may also indicate a potential kidney problem.

2. Swelling: Swelling in the face, hands, feet, and ankles can be a sign of kidney disease. This is caused by fluid retention, which is caused by an accumulation of waste products in the body due to poor kidney function.

3. Fatigue: Fatigue is a common symptom of kidney disease and is caused by anemia, which is a lack of red blood cells. Anemia is caused by inadequate production of the hormone erythropoietin, which is produced in the kidneys.

4. Itching: Itching is another symptom of kidney disease, which is caused by an accumulation of waste products in the blood.

5. Nausea and Vomiting: Nausea and vomiting may also be a sign of kidney

disease. This is caused by an accumulation of waste products in the body and can be a sign of serious kidney damage.

6. Muscle Cramps: Muscle cramps may also be a sign of kidney disease. This is caused by an accumulation of waste products in the body and can lead to muscle twitching, cramping, and pain.

7. Skin Rashes: Skin rashes may also be a sign of kidney disease. This is caused by an accumulation of waste products in the body, which can lead to an itchy, red, and scaly rash.

These are some of the most common symptoms of kidney disease. If you experience any of these symptoms, it is important to see a doctor as soon as possible. Early diagnosis and treatment of kidney disease can help prevent or slow further damage to the kidneys and improve overall health.

Chapter 2: Understanding Chronic Kidney Disease

Diagnosis of Chronic Kidney Disease

The diagnosis of CKD involves a number of tests, including a physical exam, blood tests, and imaging tests. During the physical exam, the doctor will check the patient's blood pressure, heart rate, and look for signs of swelling in the body. Blood tests are used to measure the levels of creatinine, urea, and other substances in the blood that may indicate a kidney problem. Imaging tests, such as ultrasounds, CT scans, and MRIs, are used to look at the structure of the kidneys and any blockages or abnormalities that may be present.

The most common test used to diagnose CKD is a urinalysis. This test measures the levels of substances, such as proteins and salts, in the urine. A high level of these substances may be an indication of CKD. In addition, a urine sample may be used to measure the amount of creatinine, which is a waste product normally excreted by the kidneys. A high level of creatinine in the urine can be a sign of impaired kidney function.

Another test that may be used to diagnose CKD is a glomerular filtration rate (GFR) test. This test measures how quickly the kidneys can filter waste products from the blood. A low GFR result may indicate CKD.

CKD can also be diagnosed through other tests, such as a kidney biopsy and a renal angiogram. A biopsy is a procedure in which a small piece of tissue is taken from the kidney to be examined under a microscope. A renal angiogram is an imaging test that looks at the blood vessels in the kidneys.

Once CKD has been diagnosed, the doctor will recommend a treatment plan. Treatment typically includes lifestyle changes, medications, and, in some cases, dialysis or a kidney transplant. It is important to follow the doctor's recommendations in order to slow the progression of the disease and avoid further complications.

Treatment and Management of Chronic Kidney Disease

Treatment and management of CKD involves lifestyle changes, medications, and potentially dialysis or a kidney transplant.

Lifestyle Changes

Making lifestyle changes is one of the most important aspects of managing CKD. These changes include eating a healthy and balanced diet, maintaining a healthy weight, exercising regularly, and quitting smoking.

Eating a healthy diet can help reduce the amount of waste that the kidneys have to filter. This includes avoiding foods that are high in salt, saturated fat, and cholesterol. It is also important to limit the amount of fluids that are consumed and to stay hydrated.

Medications

Medications are also used to manage CKD. These medications can be used to treat high blood pressure, reduce protein in the urine, and prevent complications of CKD. ACE inhibitors and ARBs are often used to reduce high blood pressure, which can help slow the progression of CKD. Diuretics can also be used to reduce fluid retention and swelling in the body. Other medications, such as phosphate binders, are used to reduce the amount of phosphorus in the blood.

Dialysis and Kidney Transplant

When CKD reaches its advanced stages, dialysis or a kidney transplant may be needed. Dialysis is a treatment that uses a machine to filter waste from the blood. It is typically done three times a week and can help manage symptoms of CKD and prevent complications. A kidney transplant is a procedure in which a healthy kidney is transplanted into the body of a person with CKD. This helps to restore kidney function and can improve quality of life.

Living with CKD

Living with CKD can be difficult, but there are ways to manage the condition and improve quality of life. It is important to make lifestyle changes, take medications as prescribed, and attend regular doctor visits. By following these steps, people with CKD can help slow the progression of the disease and reduce the risk of complications.

It is also important to seek support from family and friends. Having a support system can help provide emotional support and make managing CKD easier. It is also important to seek out resources and support groups for people with CKD. This can help provide useful information and resources.

Chapter 3: Nutrition and Diet in Chronic Kidney Disease

The Basics of Nutrition and Diet in Chronic Kidney Disease

Nutrition and diet in chronic kidney disease (CKD) are important components of managing the condition. Proper nutrition and diet help to limit the progression of CKD, alleviate symptoms, and improve overall health. Nutrition and diet can also help to reduce the risk of complications, including cardiovascular disease.

The diet for those with CKD should be tailored to the individual's needs, based on the stage of the disease, lab values, and other factors. Generally, a diet that is low in sodium, potassium, and phosphorus is recommended. It is also important to maintain adequate protein intake and limit saturated and trans fats.

For those with CKD, it is important to monitor intake of essential vitamins and minerals, such as vitamin D, calcium, magnesium, iron, and zinc. These micronutrients are important for overall health and for preventing complications.

It is also important to monitor fluid intake for those with CKD. Too much fluid can cause fluid overload and lead to complications. The goal is to maintain a balance between fluid intake and output.

It is also important to monitor physical activity for those with CKD. Regular exercise helps to maintain muscle strength, flexibility, and balance.

Overall, nutrition and diet in chronic kidney disease are important components of managing the condition. A diet that is tailored to the individual's needs is important for maintaining overall health and preventing complications. It is also important to monitor intake of essential vitamins and minerals, fluid intake, and physical activity. Together, these components can help to slow the progression of CKD and improve overall health.

Low Sodium Diet

Chronic kidney disease (CKD) is a progressive condition that can cause permanent damage to the kidneys over time and is associated with a range of health problems. Proper nutrition and diet are essential for managing CKD and reducing its progression. A low-sodium diet is recommended for people with CKD, as high sodium intake can worsen the condition.

Sodium is an essential mineral, and the body needs a certain amount to maintain normal bodily functions, such as maintaining the balance of fluids and electrolytes. However, too much sodium can be detrimental to health, especially for people with CKD. Excess sodium can cause fluid retention and high blood pressure, both of which can worsen kidney function. It can also increase the risk of cardiovascular problems, such as heart attack and stroke. Therefore, it is important for people with CKD to follow a low-sodium diet.

A low-sodium diet is one that contains less than 2,000 mg of sodium per day. This is considerably lower than the recommended amount for the general population, which is no more than 2,300 mg per day. To reduce sodium intake, it is important to read nutrition labels on food products and choose items that are low in sodium. It is also beneficial to limit processed and prepared foods, as these often contain high amounts of sodium.

In addition to reducing sodium intake, a healthy diet for people with CKD should include foods that are rich in essential nutrients, such as proteins, vitamins, and minerals. Protein is especially important, as it helps to maintain muscle mass, which can slow the progression of CKD. Good sources of protein include lean meats, fish, eggs, and dairy products. It is also important to get enough vitamins and minerals from fruits and vegetables, as well as whole grains.

It is important to drink plenty of fluids every day to help flush out toxins from the body and keep the kidneys healthy. Water is the best choice for hydration, as it does not contain any sodium.

A low-sodium diet is essential for people with CKD. It is important to reduce sodium intake by reading nutrition labels and limiting processed and prepared foods. It is also beneficial to consume plenty of proteins, vitamins, and minerals from healthy sources such as lean meats, fish, eggs, dairy, fruits, vegetables, and whole grains. Finally, it is important to drink enough fluids every day to help flush out toxins and keep the kidneys healthy.

Low Potassium Diet

Chronic kidney disease (CKD) is a condition in which the kidneys are no longer able to perform their normal function of filtering and removing waste from the body. It is a progressive condition that can lead to end-stage renal disease (ESRD), which requires dialysis or a kidney transplant to maintain life.

Nutrition and diet play a major role in managing CKD. People with CKD are advised to consume a balanced diet that is low in salt, protein, phosphorus, and potassium. A low potassium diet is especially important for those with CKD because it helps to control blood levels of potassium, a mineral that can accumulate in the body and cause serious health problems.

When it comes to potassium, foods are generally divided into two categories: high-potassium foods and low-potassium foods. High-potassium foods include bananas, potatoes, and spinach, while low-potassium foods include apples, white rice, and most dairy products. People with CKD should avoid eating too many high-potassium foods and focus on consuming more low-potassium foods.

In addition to avoiding high-potassium foods, people with CKD should also limit their intake of some other foods. These include processed foods, foods high in sodium, and foods with added sugar. It may also be necessary to limit or avoid caffeine and alcohol.

Finally, it is important to stay hydrated by drinking plenty of fluids. Dehydration can worsen CKD symptoms, so it is important to drink enough fluids to prevent dehydration.

Nutrition and diet are important components of managing CKD. A balanced diet that is low in potassium, sodium, and added sugar can help to keep symptoms under control and reduce the risk of complications. It is also important to stay hydrated by drinking plenty of fluids. By following these dietary tips, people with CKD can improve their health and quality of life.

Low Phosphorous Diet

Phosphorus is an essential mineral that is found in many foods, including dairy, grains, and meats. It is important for cell growth, energy production, and bone health. However, in CKD, phosphorus can build up in the blood and cause complications. A low phosphorus diet helps to maintain healthy levels of phosphorus in the blood, while providing the essential nutrients needed for overall health.

When following a low phosphorus diet, it is important to limit foods that are high in phosphorus, such as dairy, meat, and grains. Instead, focus on eating foods that are low in phosphorus, such as fruits, vegetables, and legumes. It is also important to include foods that are high in calcium to help balance out the phosphorus. This can include dairy products that are low in phosphorus, such as cheeses and yogurt.

It is also important to limit foods that are high in sodium, as sodium can increase the amount of phosphorus in the body. This includes processed and fast foods, as well as canned and packaged foods. Additionally, it is important to limit the intake of alcohol, as it can also increase phosphorus levels.

It is important to talk to a healthcare provider or a dietitian to develop a meal plan that is tailored to your individual needs. They will be able to provide guidance on what foods are low in phosphorus, as well as help to create a meal plan that meets your nutritional needs.

A low phosphorus diet is beneficial for patients with chronic kidney disease. It helps to maintain healthy levels of phosphorus in the blood, while providing the essential nutrients needed for overall health. It is important to talk to a healthcare provider or dietitian to develop an individualized meal plan that meets your nutritional needs.

Low Protein Diet

A low-protein diet is often recommended for people with CKD, as high-protein diets can increase the workload on the kidneys and worsen the condition.

A low-protein diet should be tailored to the individual's needs. Generally, the diet should provide enough protein to meet the body's requirements while avoiding excessive amounts. A dietitian can help in designing a meal plan that meets the patient's individual needs. People with CKD should also strive to maintain a healthy weight and avoid excessive sodium intake.

Foods to include in a low-protein diet for people with CKD include fruits and vegetables, whole grains, legumes, nuts and seeds, and low-fat dairy products. These foods provide essential vitamins and minerals while also providing a source of energy. It is important to note that while limiting protein intake is important, it is also important to get enough of the essential amino acids that are found in protein. These essential amino acids can be obtained from plant-based proteins such as beans, lentils, nuts, and seeds.

In addition to eating a balanced diet, people with CKD should also drink plenty of fluids to prevent dehydration. Dehydration can lead to an increase in urea and creatinine levels, which can further worsen the condition.

Nutrition and diet play an important role in managing CKD. It is important for people with CKD to work with a dietitian to ensure that their meal plan is tailored to their individual needs. A low-protein diet can help to reduce the workload on the kidneys and slow the progression of CKD. Eating a balanced diet, including plenty of fruits and vegetables, whole grains, legumes, nuts and seeds, and low-fat dairy products, while avoiding excess sodium and maintaining a healthy weight can help to improve overall health and well-being.

The exact amount of protein that should be restricted depends on the individual's kidney function and other risk factors.

Generally, the recommended daily protein intake for people with CKD is 0.6-0.8 grams of protein per kilogram of body weight. For example, a person who weighs 70 kg (154 lbs) should aim to consume between 42-56 grams of protein per day.

In addition to restricting protein intake, it is important to ensure that the types of protein consumed are of high quality. Animal proteins such as meat, fish, and eggs contain all the essential amino acids that our bodies need, and are therefore the best sources of protein for someone with CKD. Plant proteins such as legumes, nuts, and seeds should also be included in the diet, but they should be combined with other plant proteins to ensure that all essential amino acids are consumed.

It is important to note that a low-protein diet does not mean a low-calorie diet. People with CKD should still consume enough calories to meet their energy needs, as a low-calorie diet can lead to further health problems.

When following a low-protein diet, it is also important to make sure that you are getting enough vitamins and minerals. People with CKD may need to take supplements to ensure that they are getting enough of these important nutrients.

In summary, a low-protein diet is an important dietary intervention for people with CKD. It can help to reduce the workload on the kidneys and reduce the amount of waste products that can accumulate in the blood. It is important to ensure that the types of protein consumed are of high quality and that enough calories are consumed to meet energy needs. Finally, it is important to ensure that enough vitamins and minerals are consumed to meet nutritional needs.

Fluid Restriction

Fluid restriction is an important part of the nutrition plan for those with CKD. This means that individuals with CKD need to limit their intake of fluids to an amount that is safe for their kidneys to handle. Depending on the stage of their CKD, individuals may need to restrict their fluid intake to between 500 and 1500 ml per day. This can be a difficult adjustment to make, as it requires limiting a wide range of foods and beverages, including some of the most popular drinks, such as soda and fruit juice.

When it comes to fluid restriction, it is important to understand why it is necessary. When the kidneys are not functioning properly, they cannot effectively remove excess fluids from the body. This can lead to an accumulation of fluids in the body, which can cause a wide range of symptoms, such as swelling, high blood pressure, and an increased risk of heart failure. By limiting fluid intake, individuals with CKD can reduce the burden on their kidneys and help to prevent these symptoms from occurring.

It is also important to note that fluid restriction does not mean eliminating all fluids from the diet. Instead, it is important to choose fluids that are low in sodium and high in potassium, such as water, low-sodium vegetable juices, and herbal teas. Additionally, individuals with CKD should avoid coffee, alcohol, and sugary drinks, as these can further increase the risk of complications.

Fluid restriction is an important part of the nutrition plan for those with chronic kidney disease. This means limiting the amount of fluids consumed to an amount that is safe for the kidneys to handle. This can involve limiting a wide range of foods and drinks, including some of the most popular beverages, such as soda and fruit juice. Additionally, it is important to choose fluids that are low in sodium and high in potassium, such as water, low-sodium vegetable juices, and herbal teas. By following a fluid restriction plan, individuals with CKD can reduce the burden on their kidneys and help to prevent the development of further complications.

Chapter 4: Recipes for Chronic Kidney Disease

Breakfast Recipes

Breakfast is the most important meal of the day and it should be full of nutrients, especially if you are dealing with chronic kidney disease. Eating healthy can help you manage your kidney disease and reduce the risk of further complications. Here are some breakfast recipes for chronic kidney disease that can be tailored to meet your needs:

Oatmeal with Fruit:

Practical Steps on how to prepare Oatmeal with Fruit

1. Gather your ingredients. You will need oatmeal, milk, water, honey, cinnamon, and your favorite fruit.

2. Measure 1/2 cup of oatmeal, 1 cup of milk, and 1 cup of water into a pot.

3. Put the pot onto the stove and bring the mixture to a boil while stirring occasionally.

4. Turn the heat down to low and simmer for 5 minutes, stirring occasionally.

5. Add honey and cinnamon to taste.

6. Remove the oatmeal from the heat and transfer it to a bowl.

7. Top with your favorite fruit.

8. Enjoy!

Scrambled Eggs with Vegetables: Scrambled eggs are a great source of protein and can be combined with a variety of vegetables for a nutrient-dense meal. Try adding in spinach, tomatoes, mushrooms, or bell peppers for an easy and delicious breakfast.

Practical Steps on how to prepare Scrambled Eggs with Vegetables

1. Start by gathering your ingredients. You will need eggs, vegetables of your choice (such as peppers, onions, mushrooms, tomatoes, etc.), butter or oil, salt, and pepper.

2. Chop the vegetables into small pieces.

3. Heat the butter or oil in a pan over medium heat.

4. Add the vegetables to the pan and sauté them until they are soft.

5. Crack the eggs into a bowl and whisk them until fluffy.

6. Add the eggs to the pan and stir everything together.

7. Season with salt and pepper to taste.

8. Continue stirring until the eggs are cooked to your desired doneness.

9. Serve the scrambled eggs with vegetables and enjoy!

Smoothie Bowl: Smoothie bowls are a great way to get in a variety of nutrients in a single meal. Start with a banana or other fruit, add a scoop of nut butter, and top it with a variety of seeds and nuts. Add a scoop of protein powder or Greek yogurt if desired.

Practical Steps on how to prepare Smoothie Bowl

1. Gather the ingredients: Start by gathering all the ingredients you'll need for your smoothie bowl. You'll need a base such as almond milk or yogurt, fresh or frozen fruit, some type of liquid sweetener (like honey or agave nectar), and optional extras like nuts, seeds, and/or protein powder.

2. Prep the ingredients: If you're using fresh fruit, wash and chop it up before adding it to the blender. If you're using frozen fruit, make sure it's thawed out before adding it to the blender.

3. Blend the ingredients: Start by adding the base (almond milk or yogurt) to the blender, then add in the fruit, liquid sweetener, and optional extras. Blend everything together until it's a smooth and creamy consistency.

4. Pour the smoothie into a bowl: Once everything is blended, pour the smoothie into a bowl.

5. Add toppings: Now it's time to get creative! Add your favorite toppings such as granola, nuts, seeds, fresh fruit, coconut flakes, chocolate chips, etc.

6. Enjoy! Now it's time to sit back, relax, and enjoy your delicious smoothie

Yogurt Parfait: This is an easy and delicious breakfast that can be tailored to your dietary needs. Start with a layer of plain yogurt, top it with fresh fruit, and then add a sprinkle of granola or nuts.

Practical Steps on how to prepare Yogurt Parfait

1. Gather the ingredients: Choose your favorite yogurt (plain or flavored), granola, fruits (fresh or frozen), and any other toppings you would like such as nuts, coconut flakes, chocolate chips, and honey.

2. Prepare the granola: Make sure to pre-bake the granola if you are using store-bought. You can also make your own with oats, nuts, and honey or maple syrup.

3. Cut the fruit: Slice the fresh fruit into small pieces or thaw and drain the frozen fruit.

4. Layer the ingredients: Start by putting a layer of yogurt on the bottom of the cup or jar. Then add a layer of granola, followed by a layer of fruit. Repeat the layers until the cup or jar is full.

5. Add toppings: Sprinkle your favorite toppings on top and don't forget to drizzle with honey or maple syrup.

6. Serve and enjoy: Serve your yogurt parfait immediately or store it in the fridge for later. Enjoy!

Rice Cakes with Nut Butter: Rice cakes are a great source of complex carbohydrates and can be a satisfying breakfast when topped with nut butter. For added flavor, top with a sprinkle of cinnamon or a few slices of banana.

Practical Steps on how to prepare Rice Cakes with Nut Butter

1. Preheat your oven to 350 degrees Fahrenheit.

2. Grease a baking sheet with butter or non-stick cooking spray.

3. Combine 1 cup of cooked white or brown rice, 1 egg, and 2 tablespoons of melted butter in a bowl.

4. Mix the ingredients together until they are fully combined.

5. Take a spoonful of the mixture and use your hands to form it into a patty shape.

6. Place the patties onto the greased baking sheet.

7. Bake in the preheated oven for 15 to 20 minutes.

8. Remove the rice cakes from the oven and let them cool for a few minutes.

9. Spread a tablespoon of your favorite nut butter on top of each rice cake.

10. Enjoy your freshly prepared rice cakes with nut butter!

Breakfast Burrito: Start with a whole wheat wrap, add scrambled eggs, cooked beans, and a variety of vegetables. Top with shredded cheese and hot sauce for an easy and delicious breakfast burrito.

Practical Steps On How To Prepare Breakfast Burrito

1. Preheat the oven to 350 degrees Fahrenheit (177 degrees Celsius).

2. Warm a large tortilla in the microwave for about 10 seconds.

3. Spread a thin layer of refried beans over the tortilla.

4. Add cooked scrambled eggs and cooked sausage.

5. Top with a sprinkle of cheese.

6. Fold the edges of the tortilla over the filling and roll into a burrito.

7. Place the burrito on a greased baking sheet.

8. Bake for 10 minutes.

9. Serve with salsa, if desired.

Lunch Recipes

Lunch time is an important time of day for people with chronic kidney disease (CKD). Eating a nutritious and balanced meal can help to maintain your health and manage your CKD. Here are some easy and delicious lunch recipes that are suitable for people with CKD.

Turkey and Avocado Wrap:
This wrap is a great lunch option that is full of protein, healthy fats and fiber.

1. Preheat the oven to 350°F.

2. Place the turkey slices in a shallow baking dish.

3. Drizzle the turkey slices with olive oil and season with salt and pepper.

4. Bake in the preheated ovenfor 20 minutes, flipping the slices halfway through.

5. Meanwhile, prepare the avocado by slicing it into thin slices.

6. Warm the tortillas in a pan over medium heat for 1 minute on each side.

7. Place one tortilla on a plate and layer the turkey slices and avocado slices onto the tortilla.

8. Drizzle with your favorite sauce or dressing.

9. Roll up the wrap, cut it in half and enjoy!

Tuna Salad Sandwich:
Practical Steps On How To Prepare Tuna Salad Sandwich

1. Begin by preparing the tuna salad. Drain one can of tuna and place it in a bowl.

2. Add mayonnaise, diced onion, diced celery, and pepper to the tuna. Stir until all ingredients are mixed.

3. Toast two slices of bread.

4. Spread the tuna salad on one slice of bread and top it with the other slice.

5. Cut the sandwich in half and enjoy.

Vegetarian Bean Burrito:

Practical Steps On How To Prepare Vegetarian Bean Burrito

1. Gather the necessary ingredients:

-Tortillas
-Refried beans
-Shredded cheese
-Sour cream
-Chopped tomatoes
-Shredded lettuce
-Chopped onions
-Chopped green peppers
-Salsa

2. Preheat the oven to 375 degrees Fahrenheit.

3. Spread the refried beans onto the tortillas.

4. Sprinkle the shredded cheese on top of the beans.

5. Place the tortillas on a baking sheet and bake in the preheated oven for 8-10 minutes, or until the cheese is melted and bubbly.

6. Meanwhile, prepare the toppings. Chop the tomatoes, lettuce, onions, and peppers.

7. Once the burritos are done baking, let them cool for a few minutes before adding the toppings.

8. Serve the burritos with the toppings and salsa. Enjoy!

Quinoa and Black Bean Salad:

This delicious salad is full of protein and fiber. Start by cooking one cup of quinoa according to package instructions. Once cooked, fluff with a fork and let cool. In a separate bowl, mix together one-quarter cup of cooked black beans, one-quarter cup of diced bell pepper, one-quarter cup of diced onion, one tablespoon of lemon juice and one tablespoon of olive oil. Add the cooled quinoa to the bowl and mix together. Top with a handful of baby spinach leaves and enjoy.

Veggie Sandwich

Practical Steps On How To Prepare Veggie Sandwich

1. Gather your ingredients. You will need bread, a spread (such as cream cheese, hummus, or vegan mayonnaise), vegetables of your choice (such as tomatoes, cucumbers, lettuce, sprouts, peppers, onions, etc.), and any additional toppings (such as cheese, avocado slices, olives, etc.).

2. Prepare the vegetables. Wash and slice the vegetables as desired.

3. Toast the bread. Toast the bread in a toaster or in a skillet on the stove top.

4. Spread the spread. Spread the spread of your choice on each slice of toasted bread.

5. Add the vegetables. Place the vegetables on one slice of bread.

6. Add the toppings. Place the additional toppings on the other slice of bread.

7. Assemble the sandwich. Place the top slice of bread on top of the bottom slice, with the toppings and vegetables in between.

8. Enjoy! Cut the sandwich in half and enjoy your veggie sandwich.

Dinner Recipes

1. Baked Salmon and Veggies: Preheat oven to 350 degrees. Arrange 4 (4-oz) salmon filets on a lightly greased baking sheet. Top with 1/4 cup lemon juice and 1/4 teaspoon of salt. Bake for 15 minutes. Meanwhile, toss 1 chopped zucchini, 1/2 cup sliced mushrooms, and 1/2 cup chopped bell pepper in a bowl with 1 teaspoon of olive oil. Spread the vegetables on a separate lightly greased baking sheet and bake for 10-15 minutes, until vegetables are tender.

2. Turkey and Rice Skillet: Heat 1 teaspoon of olive oil in a large skillet over medium heat. Add 1 pound of ground turkey and cook until browned, about 10 minutes. Add 1/2 teaspoon of garlic powder, 1/2 teaspoon of onion powder, 1/2 teaspoon of black pepper, 1/2 teaspoon of paprika, and 1/2 cup of chicken broth. Simmer until liquid has reduced, about 5 minutes. Add 1 cup of cooked white rice and 1/4 cup of sliced

green onions. Cook for 2-3 minutes, until heated through.

3. Butternut Squash Soup: Heat 1 teaspoon of olive oil in a large pot over medium-high heat. Add 1 diced onion, 1 diced carrot, and 1 diced celery stalk. Cook for 5 minutes. Add 4 cups of cubed butternut squash and 1/2 teaspoon of salt. Cook for 5 minutes. Add 4 cups of vegetable broth and bring to a boil. Reduce heat and simmer for 20 minutes. Puree the soup in a blender until smooth. Return to pot and heat for 5 minutes. Add 1/4 teaspoon of black pepper and 1/4 teaspoon of ground nutmeg. Serve warm.

4. Quinoa and Chickpea Bowl: Heat 1 teaspoon of olive oil in a large skillet over medium heat. Add 1/2 cup of chopped onion and cook for 5 minutes. Add 1/2 teaspoon of garlic powder, 1/2 teaspoon of ground cumin, 1/2 teaspoon of ground coriander, and 1/4 teaspoon of salt. Cook for 1 minute. Add 1 cup of cooked quinoa, 1 (15-oz) can of

chickpeas (drained and rinsed), and 1/2 cup of chopped cherry tomatoes. Cook for 5 minutes. Serve with 1/4 cup of crumbled feta cheese.

5. Baked Sweet Potato Fries: Preheat oven to 425 degrees. Slice 3 sweet potatoes into strips. Place on a baking sheet lined with parchment paper. Drizzle with 2 tablespoons of olive oil and 1/4 teaspoon of salt. Toss to coat. Bake for 15 minutes. Flip fries and bake for an additional 10 minutes, until golden brown. Serve with your favorite dipping sauce.

6. Vegetable Stir-Fry: Heat 1 teaspoon of sesame oil in a large skillet over medium heat. Add 1/2 cup of chopped onion and 1/2 cup of sliced bell peppers. Cook for 5 minutes. Add 1/2 cup of broccoli florets and 1/2 cup of sliced mushrooms. Cook for 5 minutes. Add 1/4 cup of low-sodium soy sauce and 1 tablespoon of honey. Simmer for 5 minutes. Serve over cooked brown rice.

7. Eggplant Parmesan: Preheat oven to 375 degrees. Slice 1 eggplant into 1/4-inch thick slices. Place on a baking sheet lined with parchment paper. Drizzle with 2 tablespoons of olive oil and sprinkle with 1/4 teaspoon of salt. Bake for 15 minutes. Flip eggplant slices and bake for an additional 10 minutes. Meanwhile, heat 1 teaspoon of olive oil in a large skillet over medium heat. Add 1/2 cup of chopped onion and 1/4 teaspoon of salt. Cook for 5 minutes. Add 1 (15-oz) can of no-salt-added diced tomatoes and 1 teaspoon of Italian seasoning. Simmer for 10 minutes. Layer eggplant slices in a greased baking dish. Top with tomato sauce and 1/2 cup of shredded mozzarella cheese. Bake for 10 minutes. Serve with cooked whole-wheat pasta.

8. Baked Cod with Tomatoes and Olives: Preheat oven to 400 degrees. Arrange 4 (4-oz) cod filets on a lightly greased baking sheet. Top with 1/4 cup of low-sodium

tomato sauce, 1/4 cup of sliced black olives, and 1/4 teaspoon of dried oregano. Bake for 15 minutes. Meanwhile, heat 1 teaspoon of olive oil in a small skillet over medium heat. Add 1/2 cup of chopped onion and 1/4 teaspoon of salt. Cook for 5 minutes. Add 1/2 cup of chopped cherry tomatoes and cook for 2 minutes, until heated through. Serve baked cod with onion and tomato mixture.

Snack Recipes

1. Apple and Cheese Snack: Slice an apple into thin slices and top with a slice of your favorite cheese.

2. Banana and Peanut Butter Wrap: Spread a light layer of peanut butter on a whole-wheat wrap, top with banana slices, and roll up.

3. Celery and Hummus: Spread hummus on celery sticks and enjoy.

4. Yogurt Parfait: Layer low-fat Greek yogurt with fresh berries and a sprinkle of granola for a tasty treat.

5. Trail Mix: Combine nuts, dried fruits, and whole grain cereal for a healthy snack.

6. Hard-boiled Eggs: Boil eggs the night before for an easy snack.

7. Fruit Salad: Toss together your favorite fruits for a colorful snack.

8. Popcorn: Pop a few cups of popcorn and top with a light sprinkle of Parmesan cheese.

9. Avocado Toast: Toast a piece of whole wheat bread and top with mashed avocado.

10. Veggie Chips: Bake thinly sliced carrots, sweet potatoes, or beets for a healthy and crunchy snack.

11. Cottage Cheese and Fruit: Top low-fat cottage cheese with fresh fruit for a protein-packed snack.

12. Smoothie: Blend a banana, almond milk, almond butter, and a scoop of protein powder for a quick and delicious snack.

13. Protein Shake: Blend a scoop of protein powder with milk and your favorite fruit for a filling snack.

Dessert Recipes

1. Caramelized Apple Crisp
Ingredients:
- 4 small apples, peeled and chopped
- 2 tablespoons butter
- 2 tablespoons light brown sugar
- 1 teaspoon ground cinnamon
- 1/4 teaspoon ground nutmeg
- 1/2 cup rolled oats
- 1/4 cup all-purpose flour
- 1/4 cup chopped almonds
Instructions:

1. Preheat oven to 375°F.

2. In a medium bowl, combine apples, butter, sugar, cinnamon, and nutmeg. Mix until apples are evenly coated.

3. In a separate bowl, mix together oats, flour, and almonds.

4. Spread apples in an even layer in a 9-inch baking dish. Sprinkle oat mixture over the top.

5. Bake in preheated oven for 25-30 minutes, or until apples are tender and topping is golden brown.

2. Coconut Milk Pudding
Ingredients:
- 1 can coconut milk
- 2 tablespoons cornstarch
- 2 tablespoons honey
- 1 teaspoon vanilla extract
- 1/4 teaspoon ground nutmeg
Instructions:

1. In a medium saucepan, whisk together coconut milk, cornstarch, honey, vanilla, and nutmeg.

2. Place saucepan over medium heat and cook, stirring constantly, until mixture thickens, about 5 minutes.

3. Pour pudding into individual serving dishes and let cool before serving.

3. Chocolate Avocado Mousse
Ingredients:
- 1 ripe avocado, peeled and pitted
- 1/4 cup cocoa powder
- 3 tablespoons honey
- 2 tablespoons almond milk
- 1/2 teaspoon vanilla extract
Instructions:
1. In a blender or food processor, combine avocado, cocoa powder, honey, almond milk, and vanilla. Blend or process until smooth.

2. Scoop mousse into individual serving dishes and chill for at least 30 minutes before serving.

4. Baked Apples
Ingredients:

- 4 apples, cored
- 2 tablespoons honey
- 1 teaspoon ground cinnamon
- 1/4 teaspoon ground nutmeg
- 1/4 cup chopped walnuts
Instructions:
1. Preheat oven to 350°F.
2. Place apples in a baking dish.
3. Drizzle honey over apples and sprinkle with cinnamon and nutmeg.
4. Top with chopped walnuts.
5. Bake for 20-25 minutes, or until apples are tender. Serve warm.

Conclusion

This book has shown that eating a healthy diet is an important part of managing chronic kidney disease. Through the use of simple, easy-to-follow recipes and helpful tips, this cookbook has enabled readers to create delicious and nutritious meals that help them to manage their kidney disease.

The recipes in this cookbook have been designed to help those with chronic kidney disease navigate the complexities of eating healthy and managing their condition. In addition to the recipes, the book includes information on the nutritional needs of those with kidney disease, as well as helpful tips on how to adjust one's diet to meet their individual needs.

Overall, this cookbook has provided readers with a wide variety of delicious and nutritious meal options that are specifically tailored to help them manage their chronic kidney disease. With this cookbook, readers can easily prepare meals that are not only delicious, but that also provide the essential nutrients their bodies need. By following the recipes and tips provided in this cookbook, readers can take an active role in managing their chronic kidney disease, while still enjoying delicious and healthy meals. With this cookbook, readers have been given the tools to live a healthy lifestyle, while still enjoying delicious and nutritious meals.

9 798376 656679

These ideas can help you to build a strong connection with your partner and develop a deeper understanding of them.

❖ Show appreciation: Showing appreciation for your partner can help to create a strong bond between you. Express your gratitude for the small things they do, and let them know how much you care.

❖ Communicate openly: Communication is critical in any relationship. Make sure you listen to your partner and share your thoughts and feelings openly. This can help you to build trust and understanding in your relationship.

❖ Be positive: Focusing on the positives in your relationship can help to manifest true love. Always focus on the good and avoid negative thoughts and feelings.

❖ Spend quality time together: Make sure you take the time to bond with your partner. Make enduring memories by spending time with one another.

The Power of Positive Thinking is essential for manifesting one true love. Focus on the positives in your relationship and use the tips above. You can create a strong and lasting connection with your partner. Positive thinking allows you to find the love you deserve and create a beautiful and lasting relationship.

How to Stay Connected

As we move through life, it can be easy to lose sight of what truly matters in our relationships. We can become so focused on our work, our hobbies, and our daily tasks that we forget to nurture the one true love that underlies it all.

That is why staying connected with the ones we love is so important, even when it seems like we don't have the time or resources to do so.

One of the best ways to stay connected with the one we love is through communication. We should take time daily to talk with our partners in person or over the phone. Communication keeps us connected and helps us express our feelings and understand each other better. We should also listen to our partners and how they feel—taking the time to listen to shows that we care and helps to deepen our connection.

Another way to stay connected is to make time for special activities together. Going on a date, having a weekend vacation, spending time at home, and doing something special for each other are examples demonstrating that you are still involved in the relationship.

We should also make sure to carve out time for ourselves so that we don't get too overwhelmed with the demands of everyday life. This will help us stay connected in the long run.

Finally, we should show our appreciation for each other. You can do this through small gestures such as sending a gift, writing a note, or even telling your partner how much you love and appreciate them. This will remind them how much we care and help keep our relationship strong.

By maintaining a connection with our partner, we can ensure that our relationship remains strong and vibrant. Taking the time to communicate, do special activities together, and show appreciation for each other will help keep the one true love alive in our relationship.

Chapter 2: Understanding True Love

Love is a feeling that can be difficult to explain and understand. Many people believe true love can only be felt and never truly expressed. The concept of true love has been around since ancient times and is still a hot topic today. This chapter will explore the many aspects of true love and how to recognize it when it appears.

First, let's look at the different types of love. There is the romantic love that we often associate with relationships, and there is also platonic love which is more of a friendship-based kind of love. Both of these types of love are important and have their unique qualities.

True love is more profound than either of these two types.

It is a connection between two people based on trust, respect, and a genuine appreciation for one another.

True love is not based on physical attraction, although it can be enhanced by it. It is more of an emotional connection that goes beyond the physical. It is an unbreakable bond between two people and can stand the test of time. It is a feeling that is so powerful that it can bring two people together in a way that no other emotion can.

Understanding True Love

Once you have found someone you think might be the right person for you, it is essential to understand true love. True love is not just a feeling but also a conscious choice to commit to someone and to be there for them no matter what. It requires sacrifice and unconditional acceptance of one another's flaws and imperfections.

True love is an emotional bond between two people that one cannot replicate. It is a connection built through shared experiences and mutual understanding. True love is patient, kind, and forgiving. It is a bond that is based on trust and respect.

True love is also unconditional and selfless. It is focused on the needs of the other person and not just on one's desires. It is an emotion you can feel in every moment, and it can be cherished and celebrated even in the darkest of times.

Finally, it is essential to remember that true love can be challenging. It requires hard work, dedication, and commitment to make it last. But two people are willing to put in the effort and are open to understanding one another. In that case, true love can be a gratifying experience.

What is True Love?

True love is an emotion that is often sought after but rarely experienced. It is an emotion that transcends physical attraction and forms a bond between two people that cannot be replicated. True love is a deep and meaningful connection that is not based on superficial things, such as physical appearance or wealth. It cannot be forced but must be discovered through shared experiences and mutual understanding.

True love is compassionate, patient, and forgiving. It is a connection based on trust and respect. True love is not just a feeling but also a conscious choice to commit to someone and to be there for them no matter what. It requires sacrifice and unconditional acceptance of one another's flaws and imperfections.

True love is unconditional and selfless; it is a bond between two people based on mutual understanding, respect, and loyalty. It is unconditional because it is not based on expectations of perfection or on trying to manipulate the other person. It is also selfless because it focuses on the needs of the other person and not just on one's desires.

True love is enduring, and it can last a lifetime. It can be shared between two people who are deeply and passionately in love with one another. It is an emotion that can be felt in every moment and cherished and celebrated even in the darkest of times.

The Difference Between Love and Infatuation

The difference between love and infatuation can be challenging to discern. Both feelings bring about strong emotions and intense levels of attraction and desire. Many often mistake the two for one another, but there are key differences to consider when determining which feeling one is experiencing.

Infatuation is a strong and immediate emotion that often occurs in the early stages of a romantic relationship. It's a kind of intense obsession and longing brought on by physical attraction and often leads to a fantasy-like idea of the other person.

This all-consuming emotion can be incredibly exhilarating and exciting, but it can also be dangerous and lead to a distorted perception of the other person and the relationship. It is often very short-lived and starts to fade as the relationship moves into deeper and more meaningful levels.

On the other hand, love is much more than simply a feeling of intense emotion. It is a deep connection of respect, trust, and understanding. Love typically grows over time as two people get to know each other and learn to accept one another's differences. A strong bond between two people creates an environment of safety, mutual understanding, and growth. Love is not always easy, but it still provides a consistent source of comfort and support.

While the distinction between love and infatuation can be blurry at times, taking the time to analyze the feelings and emotions one is experiencing can provide a clearer picture. If a relationship is based solely on physical attraction and desire, likely, it is primarily infatuation. If, on the other hand, the relationship provides a feeling of comfort, security, and understanding, there's a good chance that it is based on a deeper form of love. As always, only you can decide what you are truly feeling.

How to Find True Love

Finding true love is not always easy, and there is no magic formula.

It is an emotion that comes from within and is found through shared experiences and a deep connection between two people. To find true love, it is important to be open to the possibility of it and to be willing to take risks.

Being upfront and truthful about your preferences for a relationship is the first step in discovering real love. Always keep in mind to ask yourself, "What sort of person do I want to be in a relationship with?" What qualities do I need to look for in a partner? Being truthful about your preferences might help you narrow your options and concentrate your search.

Once you have a better idea of what you are looking for, it is time to start looking for potential partners. There are many different ways to do this, such as through mutual friends, online dating sites, or even chance encounters.

It is essential to be open to meeting new people and getting to know them before deciding whether or not they are the right person for you.

Finally, once you have found someone you think could be the right person for you, it is crucial to take the time to get to know them. Spend time with them, talk to them, and learn more about who they are and what they are looking for in a relationship. This will help you determine if they are genuinely the right person for you.

The Importance of Compassion and Understanding

Compassion and understanding are two of the most important traits a person can possess. For many, these qualities are also the most difficult to understand and practice as we go through life, often feeling alone and misunderstood. If we just had that extra love and understanding, our lives would be easier, more meaningful, and more connected. We often fail to realize how much compassion and understanding can truly make us feel complete in our lives.

Compassion and understanding start with ourselves, which is why it is so important to have self-compassion and self-understanding.

Understanding our deepest feelings, needs and desires can give us clarity and the ability to move forward. We must learn to forgive ourselves for our mistakes, recognize our strengths and weaknesses, and recognize our limitations. As we learn to appreciate ourselves and our individual journeys, we can begin to understand and appreciate the journeys of others.

When we extend compassion and understanding to others, we invest our time and energy in building meaningful relationships, which can lead to a life of fulfilment. By being compassionate, we learn to empathize with other people's feelings, enabling us to create an environment where everyone's needs are considered and validated.

Compassion can also give us the courage to offer strength and comfort to those in need, which could have an everlasting impact on their lives.

By striving to be compassionate and understanding in our everyday lives, we are helping to create a better world. Compassion and understanding bring us closer together, enabling us to recognize our similarities instead of focusing on our differences. We can learn to accept one another for who we are and appreciate our individual journeys. Compassion and understanding can turn a negative situation into something positive, create connections where none existed before, and help us grow and learn from each other.

Compassion and understanding are powerful tools that we can use to lead a life of connection, fulfilment, and joy.

We can create meaningful relationships and lasting happiness by humbly practicing these two traits in our lives.

Chapter 3: Appreciating Togetherness in Relationships

One of the best gifts we can ever give or receive in life is the gift of togetherness. To be able to share our life and moments with someone special is truly a blessing. Even in the most difficult times, togetherness can help us through. The sense of being appreciated and understood allows us to fully understand our own emotions and those of others.

Being in a relationship involves the willingness to appreciate each other and the moments shared, no matter how difficult or chaotic they may be.

Appreciating togetherness in relationships is a key ingredient in creating and nurturing a bond between two people. It needs to be consciously cultivated as it often gets lost in the everyday hustle and bustle of life.

The appreciation of togetherness may start with simple gestures like holding hands, taking a stroll together and having a heartfelt conversation. It may also involve doing activities together, such as planning special date nights and finding time to connect in meaningful ways.

Having a ritual of appreciation is also important. This can be done in any relationship, whether with a partner, a family member, or even a close friend.

Taking the time to check in with each other and show appreciation for being together can do wonders and is an incredibly powerful way to maintain a connection.

Sharing our thoughts, feelings and dreams with each other is also an important part of expressing our appreciation for togetherness. It is needed to strengthen the bond and is a fundamental part of understanding each other on a deeper level.

Having a deep understanding of each other is what ultimately brings us closer. It is the foundation for a relationship built on trust and mutual respect. Appreciating togetherness in relationships helps us become aware of everything that brings us closer and allows us to focus on the positive aspects of the relationship. It is a source of strength and an opportunity for growth.

Appreciating togetherness in relationships is an ongoing process that ever changes and evolves as we learn to trust, understand and appreciate each other. Relationships are too precious to take for granted, and by consciously valuing togetherness, we set ourselves up to enjoy life's most precious moments.

The Benefits of Togetherness

The best things in life are those that we share with others. Whether it is through physical presence, through writing, or through the heart, being together is one of the most important things we can do as humans.

First and foremost, togetherness helps create and maintain strong bonds between people. We are social creatures, and being with someone else helps us to better connect and form meaningful relationships. Not only that, but shared experiences and activities can bring us closer to another. When we engage in activities or conversations together, we can create a deeper understanding of each other and have a platform for increased communication.

Secondly, togetherness can help us to learn new things. Whether it be learning how to cook a new dish, practicing a new sport, or discovering deeper aspects of another culture, by engaging with someone else, we can grow and expand our knowledge in ways that would be impossible alone.

Thirdly, togetherness can foster creativity. With two heads working on a project together, we come up with ideas that neither of us would have done on their own. The power of collaboration can enable us to find creative solutions to challenging problems.

Fourthly, togetherness can positively affect our mental health. Socializing can be an important part of self-care and having a supportive, loving bond with someone can lead to increased happiness and a healthier overall mindset.

Finally, togetherness can bring about a sense of belonging. Whether it is with a family, friend, or larger group, being part of something bigger than yourself can create feelings of acceptance, security, and purpose.

In conclusion, togetherness can be an incredibly powerful force in our lives. Through shared physical presence, communication, activities, and projects, we are able to create and maintain relationships, learn new things, foster creativity, improve our mental health, and feel a sense of belonging. Through togetherness we can bring out the best in each other and in ourselves.

How to Maintain a Healthy Relationship

The key to a healthy relationship is understanding that it takes work, and working together with your partner to ensure that it is a safe and healthy dynamic.

Ultimately, it is up to both partners to invest in the relationship. Here are some tips on how to maintain a healthy and happy relationship.

Communication is perhaps the most important component of any relationship. By communicating effectively and openly, couples can understand each other on a deeper level and avoid conflicts. Communication between partners should be honest, respectful, and consistent. Consistent and clear communication will help keep the relationship healthy and strong.

It's also important to show appreciation for your partner. Simple acts of appreciation can go a long way — like expressing your love verbally, writing a note, or taking a few moments to show your partner how much you care about them.

Respect is essential in any relationship. Each partner should respect the other and their individual preferences, beliefs, and boundaries. A lack of respect can diminish trust and lead to resentment in the relationship — neither of which is healthy.

In addition to communication and respect, trust is fundamental to a healthy relationship. Both partners should trust each other and be open and honest about their feelings. Deception or dishonesty can severely damage a relationship, so it's important to be upfront with your partner and make sure that you can trust them to be honest with you.

Another way to maintain a healthy relationship is to make sure that both partners are doing their share in the relationship.

This means dividing responsibilities and taking turns when it comes to tasks such as housework and financial decisions. Neglecting responsibilities can create tension in the relationship and can lead to resentment.

Finally, couples should make time for each other and devote a portion of their day to nurture their relationship. Even something as simple as talking for 15 minutes at the end of each day can help strengthen your bond and increase mutual understanding. Spending quality time together can bring couples closer and make them feel more connected.

Maintaining a healthy and happy relationship takes effort and dedication, but it can be one of the most rewarding experiences. By putting in the work and following these tips, couples can ensure that their relationship continues to thrive.

Dealing with Conflict

Relationships require a great deal of effort, but conflict can sometimes make it challenging to stay connected to each other. Dealing with conflict in relationships can be tricky, but it's necessary for the growth of individuals and the relationship itself.

When you sense tension or conflict in a relationship, it's essential to take a deep breath and reflect on the situation. This can help you be mindful of what is going on and better understand the source of the tension.

In many cases, the underlying source of conflict is a communication breakdown. This could be anything from miscommunication, to different levels of understanding, to a reaction to the other person's perspective.

It's important to talk openly and honestly with your partner to find out the root cause of the conflict.

Another critical aspect of resolving conflict is to remain open to your partner's perspective. This means being willing to listen without judgment and understanding their point of view without getting defensive. Listening to each other can help you better understand what is causing the tension and can help to foster a sense of empathy between you.

It's also important to remember to remain patient and understanding. Conflict can be complex and often takes time to resolve. It is crucial to allow yourself and your partner to vent and be heard, even if sometimes it can be difficult to hear.

Finally, it's important to be willing to compromise. It is important to remember that you are equally responsible for the relationship, and compromise can help ensure both partners are heard and feel respected. Compromise requires patience, understanding and the ability to talk openly and honestly with each other.

Dealing with conflict in relationships can be challenging, but patience and understanding can be powerful tools for strengthening the connection between you and your partner.

Remember to stay open to each other's perspectives, communicate openly, and be willing to compromise in order to make progress. With work, respect, and dedication, you can find a way to resolve the conflict and make your relationship stronger.

Chapter 4: Applying the Manifest True Love Principles to Your Relationship

Applying the "Manifest the One True Love" Principles to Your Relationship is a powerful way to create a more fulfilling, secure, and loving connection with your partner. When both individuals in the relationship embrace and practice these principles, they can experience unparalleled love that stands the test of time.

At its core, the Manifest One True Love Principles are rooted in the power of positive thinking and self-empowerment.

When you and your partner learn to tap into the power of positive thinking, your love can become stronger and more profound. This begins with cultivating an attitude of gratitude for the love in your relationship, giving the relationship its due respect and attention, and making time for each other.

Active listening is also integral to manifesting true love, as it opens the door to better communication and understanding. Showing your partner that you are listening and paying attention by mirroring their feelings and validating them is essential to creating an environment of trust and openness.

Compromise and understanding are also critical components of a successful, loving relationship.

When you and your partner can work together to reach an agreement and understand each other's perspectives, it helps to foster a sense of security, trust, and understanding.

Finally, it would help if you never overlooked the power of kindness and appreciation. Showing your partner your fondness and admiration for them helps to feed and nurture the love in your relationship. Showing empathy and compassion to your partner, even in moments of difficulty, can help to strengthen your bond with one another.

By applying the "Manifest the One True Love" Principles to your relationship, you and your partner can experience a deeper and more meaningful connection.

When both individuals in the relationship actively work to cultivate gratitude, practice active listening, compromise, and show kindness and appreciation, the relationship is sure to benefit and become more fulfilling.

The "Manifest True Love" Process

The "Manifest True Love" Process is a journey that helps to unleash your potential for personal growth and for finding true love. As you embark on this journey, you will access powerful techniques that will assist you in understanding your own and others' needs.

You will learn to recognize the signs that indicate the presence of a possible mate, and it will better equip you to create loving relationships.

The process begins with connecting to the power of "Love". When you are connected to the power of love, you will learn to recognize the feelings inside you that indicate whether you have a good connection with someone or not. This connection to the power of love will allow you to identify the qualities in a person or situation that attract you and those that you can overcome.

You will learn to understand your potential partner's needs as you move forward. You will learn the skills necessary to communicate effectively and the importance of establishing boundaries in relationships.

You will also explore how to create a balance of power between you and your potential partner.

With the Manifest the One True Love Process, you will learn to make choices that will bring you closer to finding the one true love that you crave. You will gain insight into ways to nurture and sustain the connection with your partner. You will also discover how to avoid pitfalls that often prevent successful relationships from taking shape.

You will learn how to manifest your dream relationship by consciously changing your thoughts and feelings and visualizing a positive outcome. You will discover the power of forgiveness and how it can help you move on from past relationships and move forward. You will also be taught the importance of letting go of your expectations and allowing yourself to be open to the possibilities of love.

The "Manifest the One True Love" Process is a journey that will empower you to create the kind of relationship that you desire. You will gain insight into yourself and the way that you interact with others. You will learn to recognize and embrace the magic of finding true love. The journey concludes by celebrating the power of love and its richness in your life.

How to Create a Manifest True Love Mindset

These days, it seems as though many of us are searching for true love—something real and lasting. The idea of finding "the one" can leave us feeling overwhelmed, uncertain, and hopeless.

After all, what are the chances of us finding someone who is truly perfect for us and will stay with us forever?

If you're feeling discouraged, it is time to shift your mindset. Instead of focusing on finding "the one," why not focus on creating "the one" in your own life?

Creating a mindset of manifesting your one true love begins with shifting your focus away from the idea of searching or waiting and instead embracing the power of attraction. You need to believe that true love is possible and is already coming your way. When you believe in something, the Universe will respond by sending it to you.

The next step is to create an intention for the kind of love you want to attract. Ask yourself what qualities you want in a partner and write them down.

Visualize your ideal relationship, and imagine the happy moments you will share. Create a detailed vision of the relationship you would like to have, and make sure to keep it optimistic.

With a firm intention in place, it is time to take action. You may be tempted to rush out and start dating, but be mindful that true love often takes time to develop. Instead, focus on nurturing your inner self and setting yourself up for success. Take care of yourself, spend time in activities that bring you joy, and connect with people who believe in love.

After taking action and giving the Universe time to bring your one true love to you, it is essential to stay mindful and open. Pay attention to the signs and synchronicities that come your way, and be patient and trusting that your one true love will eventually come.

Creating a mindset of manifesting your one true love involves recognizing that the power to attract your perfect partner is in your hands. By shifting your focus and embracing the power of attraction, you can confidently create an intention and take action towards meeting your one true love. So put aside doubts or fears, and take the first step on your journey to manifest the love you desire and deserve.

Tools for Manifesting the One True Love

When it comes to "manifesting the one true love", tools and strategies are essential.

The right tools can not only help you attract the right person but also help to ensure that they stay with you.

Visualization is the most common tool used by those manifesting true love. Visualization is creating a vivid mental image of what you would like your dream relationship to resemble. It could include a mental snapshot of the person you want to be with, the home you would like to share, the activities you would like to do together, and any other aspect of your relationship that you would like to manifest. It is essential to really picture the details clearly and to feel the emotions that come along with the image of your dream relationship.

Gratitude is another critical tool for manifesting true love. It is essential to cultivate a sense of appreciation for the things already showing up in your life.

This is a fundamental step in the manifesting process. It helps to ensure that you send positive energy into the universe and invite more of what you want into your life. Being thankful for the blessings you already have paves the way for you to receive even more.

The Law of Attraction is another powerful tool that can be used when manifesting true love. This tool is based on the idea that 'like attracts like.' This means that whatever energy you send into the universe will be reflected in you.

It is essential to be mindful of the thoughts that you are thinking and the beliefs that you are carrying, as these will influence the type of partner that you manifest into your life.

These are just a few of the tools and strategies that can be employed when manifesting true love.

It is essential to remember that the process only happens after a while but requires patience and practice. With the right tools and strategies in place, you will be well on your way to manifesting the one true love of your dreams.

Chapter 5: Tips for Making Valentine's Day Special

Valentine's Day is around the corner, and many people look forward to a special day of love and romance. Whether you have a significant other or are looking forward to celebrating with family and friends, making Valentine's Day special can be as easy as planning ahead. Here are some tips for making the special day a memorable one.

First and foremost, plan something fun and romantic that you and your sweetheart will enjoy. A few possibilities are a romantic dinner out, a movie, or a play.

If you need to figure out what your sweetheart would like, spend some time online or in your local store researching something special and unique. Give yourself enough time to generate ideas and make reservations if necessary.

Second, consider making your own Valentine's Day cards. Whether at home, out on a date, or going to meet up with friends, handing out homemade cards can be a sweet way to express your love and appreciation. Crafting these cards also gives you time to work out what you want to say, so you can make sure you leave a lasting impression.

Third, think about an activity that the two of you can do together. You could plan a surprise dance lesson or a cooking class.

If you don't know what your sweetheart would like, consider asking their family and friends for ideas, they may know of a hobby or activity that your special someone loves to do.

Lastly, do something special to surprise your sweetheart. If you know they love surprises, take them on a fun, romantic day trip, fill the house with roses and candles for a romantic night in, or give them a heartfelt handwritten letter that expresses how much you care about them. This will surely put a smile on their face and make them feel loved.

However, if you decide to celebrate Valentine's Day, keep in mind that it's the thought that counts. Taking the time to make your significant other feel special will show them how much you care and make the day more memorable.

You can make this Valentine's Day extra special with a little preparation and a few thoughtful gestures.

Planning a Special Date

Planning a special date is one of the most exciting and romantic things you can do with your partner. When planning the perfect date night, it's essential to consider the type of activities and décor that will make your romantic evening one to remember. From choosing the right restaurant and the perfect gift to planning the ambiance and setting, there are plenty of ways to make your special date an unforgettable experience.

When choosing a restaurant for your special date, you want to ensure it's the perfect fit for both of you. Consider your food preferences, budget, and location. You can also research restaurants online to see what types of reviews they have. Once you've chosen a restaurant, make your reservation in advance.

You also want to consider what types of gifts you'll give your special someone. A nice box of chocolates or flowers can be a great way to show appreciation. For a unique present, you can create a custom gift basket with items that reflect your partner's interests and tastes.

The décor of your special night should also reflect your shared interests. You can decorate the table with a romantic centerpiece, lit candles, and photos of the two of you together. Music can also help set the mood, so choose a great playlist tailored to your date night.

If you're going somewhere special, taking along a bottle of wine or some champagne can also be helpful to add to the romantic atmosphere.

Finally, it's essential to plan out the conversation topics. Talk about things both of you enjoy, such as current events, shared hobbies, books you've read, and anything else that comes to mind. Sharing stories about your past and discussing your plans can also help you get to know each other better. With proper planning and a little bit of creativity, you can make your special date night an unforgettable experience.

Gifting Ideas

There are endless possibilities when it comes to gifting ideas for a partner on a special occasion. Whether it is a birthday, anniversary, wedding, or another special day, a gift can be the perfect way to show appreciation and love. It is important to remember that your gift should be thoughtful and personalized. Some ideas that may suit the occasion include:

❖ Jewellery – Jewellery is a timeless gift that symbolizes your relationship and makes your partner feel extra special. Many options are available, from charm bracelets and necklaces to rings and earrings. Whether they prefer something more classic or something more on-trend, there is sure to be something suitable.

- ❖ Getaway – A getaway provides a much-needed opportunity for your partner to relax and enjoy quality time together. Consider a romantic weekend away, a staycation, or a deep dive into the local sights and attractions.

- ❖ Personalized gifts – A personalized gift is a great way to show your partner that you have honestly thought about the gift and have customized it to their taste. Consider a personalized mug, t-shirt, or cushion cover with a meaningful quote or sentiment.

- ❖ Experiences – An experience is a memorable and unique way to show your partner how much you care.

Consider a cooking class, a spa day, an adventure outing, or tickets to a show or movie.

❖ Photo albums – A well-made photo album is a beautiful way to commemorate a special trip, memorable event, or everyday moments that mean so much. Put it together in a beautiful album, and watch your partner smile as they relive the shared memories.

Whichever gift you choose, make sure that it's something unique and meaningful. After all, it's all about the thought you put into it. Show your partner how much they mean to you, and make the occasion unforgettable.

Unique Ways to Celebrate

Valentine's season is renowned for being a time of celebration, romance, and love. Every couple celebrates Valentine's Day in unique and special ways. To ensure you and your partner have a memorable day, here are some unique and creative ways to celebrate with your partner this Valentine's season!

Embark on a romantic day trip. Instead of going for the usual dinner date, take a day trip with your partner to explore a nearby city or historical site. This will give you both an opportunity to explore and enjoy something new and spend quality time together.

Write each other love letters. This is a unique way to express your love and appreciation for each other. You can either write traditional love letters or get creative and create a "love book" filled with your favorite memories or photos of the two of you.

Create a romantic dinner. Even if you can't go out for dinner, you can still recreate a restaurant ambiance in your home. Get creative and make a lavish three-course meal with a bottle of wine and the perfect music. Candles and soft lighting will help create a romantic atmosphere.

Make a time capsule. This is a great way to show your partner how much you have loved them for years. Fill a box with some meaningful items, such as photos, cards, and souvenirs. Seal the box and set a date for when to open it—it could be anything from a year to a decade!

Put on a dance performance. Learn a few dance moves and give your partner a surprise performance. Dancing is an incredibly romantic way to express your love—it's also a lot of fun!

Go stargazing. Take your partner on a romantic night out under the stars. Nothing says romance quite like a starlit night. Prepare some hot chocolate, a blanket, and lots of stars to admire.

Have a sentimental movie night. Get a projector and screen and watch your favorite romantic movie. You can also create a movie night with some of your favorite memories. Bring popcorn and your favorite candy for an extra-special movie night.

No matter what unique way you celebrate with your partner, the most important thing is to have fun and show affection for each other.

Make sure to enjoy your special Valentine's season together!

Chapter 6: Recognizing Your True Love

It is said that true love comes once in a lifetime, but many do not recognize it when it arrives. True love requires patience and understanding. It requires self-awareness and being connected to feelings, which can be a challenge. Many find themselves suddenly in the throes of a passionate romance, only to discover that it was an infatuation that quickly faded away. Conversely, true love has a solid foundation and is built upon an enduring connection.

True love stands the test of time—it is not something that fades in a few weeks or months. It is deep and enduring and develops over time through communication and shared experiences. True love is unconditional; it has no parameters and does not depend on physical attraction. It relies on mutual respect, loyalty, trust, and a desire to be with the other person. Love comes in all shapes and sizes, so you must choose wisely and feel a genuine connection with the person with whom you're together.

When you meet someone you feel a genuine connection with; it is crucial to take the time to get to know them on the deepest level. Open up and talk to them; allow yourself to be vulnerable. Inquire about them and learn what makes them tick. Share your thoughts and feelings, and be honest about your intentions.

Communicating and listening to one another builds trust, and you will be able to recognize if the love you feel is true.

When you are genuinely in love, your partner will bring out the best in you. Rather than focusing on the things you don't like about each other, you will appreciate the things that you admire. You will be inspired by one another and will bring out the best in each other. Together, you will create a strong bond that only deepens over time, and you will never want to let go.

When you find true love, you should hang onto it and cherish it. Recognizing true love can be challenging, but if you are honest with yourself and try to get to know the person you are with, it can be done.

When you find true love, it is something that should be cherished and nurtured. It will help you grow and make you a better person.

How to Identify Your Soulmate

Have you ever wondered how you can determine who your soulmate is? Finding and connecting with your soulmate can be one of the most rewarding experiences you may ever encounter during your life's journey. A soulmate is a special person who resonates with you deeply, intimately—beyond the surface level of physical attraction and personality.

However, it can be challenging to identify your soulmate, not to mention developing a relationship with them and strengthening it over time. To help here are several tips to help you determine if someone is your true soulmate.

1. Intuition: One of the most reliable ways to identify your soulmate is to tap into intuition. Much like a sixth sense, your intuition is the inner voice that can guide you when searching for the right person. Listen to what your gut tells you, and be aware of any signs or symbols coming your way.

2. Connection: When you interact with a potential soulmate, pay close attention to your connection with them. If you experience a strong bond and feel like you just "clicked", this could signify that you have found your soulmate.

Look for signs such as feeling completely comfortable and safe with them and having an instant familiarity, even if you've never met before.

3. Values Alignment: A soulmate connection is based on shared values and beliefs. When looking for your soulmate, be aware of how their values and beliefs align with yours. Your soulmate should share your most important values and support them in return.

4. Positive Energy: A soulmate connection will bring with it a strong sense of positive energy. This energy can be felt when you are in each other's presence, making you feel safe, happy, and fulfilled in the relationship.

5. Mutual Respect: Respect is an essential component of a soulmate relationship.

You should be able to respect each other's differences and appreciate them as unique individuals. Look for a strong sense of mutual respect and support to identify a potential soulmate.

Ultimately, finding a soulmate connection is a personal journey that is unique to each individual. By following these tips, you can gain clarity and insight into the process of identifying your soulmate.

The Significance of the Relationship

The relationship between individuals is essential to a meaningful life.

It shapes our outlook, experiences, and, ultimately, the person we become. The significance of a relationship is manifest in numerous ways, most notably through its impact on our psychological, physical, mental, and emotional well-being.

When individuals have the courage to open up to each other and share their stories, it can create a sense of community, belonging, and connection. It allows for feelings of security, trust, support, and understanding. A good relationship is a place of refuge and healing and can lower stress levels and anxiety.

Indeed, research has found that increased social support is associated with improved physical and psychological health, better psychological functioning, and enhanced mood.

At its core, a relationship is the sharing of mutual respect and understanding.

A successful relationship happens when there is an exchange of feelings and emotions, which enable the partners to learn more about themselves and each other, and to build a deep bond. This bond is special because it allows both people to grow and develop together, without fear or judgment. Furthermore, it allows individuals to open up and be vulnerable with each other, overcoming potential barriers to communication and strengthening the bond between them.

The significance of the relationship between individuals is further amplified when they can support each other through difficult times, both in terms of direct support and also indirect support.

Direct support may involve offering support and reassurance in times of hardship, while indirect support may involve providing sincere advice, guidance, and encouragement. This can be particularly meaningful in times of crisis and difficulty and can provide valuable comfort and understanding.

Ultimately, the significance of the relationship between individuals is tangible and all-encompassing. It is a relationship of distinct importance and value, which can lead to increased psychological, physical, mental, and emotional well-being. It is a connection that should not be taken for granted, and should instead be nourished, appreciated, and cherished.

The Benefits of Being with the One

When you find your one true love, something magical happens. You suddenly feel like you belong in the world, and you're ready to take on all of life's adventures. Being with the one you truly love gives you a sense of security that you can't find anywhere else. Your life is suddenly filled with the joy of being accepted and loved for who you are.

The benefits of being with the one true love are endless. You are no longer afraid of taking risks or facing your fears, knowing that you'll always have a partner who will be there to pick you up if you fall. You learn to appreciate the little things in life, like a warm embrace or a meaningful conversation.

Your worries and doubts melt away, replaced by a sense of confidence and purpose.

Being with the one true love means having someone to share your triumphs and misfortunes. You can count on your partner to help you make the right decisions and to offer support and understanding during difficult times. You can also take comfort in knowing that your loved one will always be there for you when you need them.

When it comes to having a healthy relationship, being with one true love is just as important as it is fulfilling. Your relationship becomes a source of strength and a symbol of commitment to each other.

Love itself is a powerful force that can transform lives when two people open themselves up to it. When there is love, there is hope, and that hope can bring about an incredible sense of peace and contentment.

The benefits of being with the one true love are immeasurable. You experience a greater appreciation for life, knowing that the person you love is always by your side. With the right person, you can find a new sense of courage and strength to face the world, and you'll never have to feel alone again.

Chapter 7: Conclusion

Personal preferences will ultimately determine the outcome. You need to be willing to work hard to maintain a successful relationship. You must be prepared to go above and beyond each day to demonstrate your love for your mate. The goal is to strike a balance between when to push and when to back off.

It takes bravery to love and be loved. True love is not always simple, but it is always worthwhile to put in the effort.

It is the most satisfying experience you can have when you find the one, the one who genuinely loves and understands you and with whom you can live your life.

Never, ever lose hope in your quest to discover your one true love. There is someone out there who will accept you for who you are and love you with all of your flaws and oddities. All you have to do is wait, be tough, and never give up on yourself. True love exists and is waiting to be discovered.

The Benefits of Manifesting the One True Love

The concept of manifestation has been around for centuries, with many ancient cultures employing the practice in various forms. Manifesting the one true love is an increasingly popular practice in the modern world because it provides powerful insights into the Law of Attraction and its application to relationships.

Manifesting the one true love is the act of visualizing and believing in the ideal partner for you. It's about envisioning a specific kind of relationship and envisioning it with a specific type of person. By setting the intention to manifest your ultimate romantic partner from the universe, you create a powerful force that paves the way for the relationship you want.

When it comes to manifesting your one true love, there are several benefits to this approach. The first advantage is that it allows you to let go of expectations and preconceived notions about relationships. It allows you to focus on the qualities you desire in a partner, rather than settling for someone based on what society expects. This helps you avoid toxic or dysfunctional relationships and instead draws you to genuine, healthy connections.

In addition, the manifestation process can help you to become more accepting of yourself and those around you. By visualizing the perfect partner for you, you become more aware of the qualities that you bring to relationships. This self-awareness and appreciation can help you to become more confident in yourself and your relationships.

Finally, manifesting the one true love enables you to bring more passion and joy into your life. This is because when you visualize and focus on your dream relationship, you become more passionate and excited about the prospect of having it in your life. This passion and enthusiasm can oftentimes attract new and exciting relationships into your life.

Overall, manifesting the one true love can be a powerful way to improve your relationships and bring more joy and passion into your life. Not only does it help you become more accepting of yourself and those around you, but it also helps you to avoid settling for less than you deserve. By embracing this approach to relationships, you can create the kind of fulfilling relationship you have always wanted.

Reflection on What You Have Learned

Manifest the One True Love, by Monica Thomas, is an insightful and highly valuable guidebook on how to create a meaningful life and lasting relationship. This book is an invaluable resource for individuals looking to create a life-long love and meaningful intimate relationship.

The book outlines a four-step journey to manifesting one true love. This journey begins with self-discovery and the exploration of what it means to be truly authentic, honest, and vulnerable. It focuses on developing the necessary tools and practices to cultivate a sense of self-awareness, self-confidence, and self-love.

Through this process, one can develop trust in themselves and their relationship with the universe.

In the second step, one begins to delve into the importance of understanding the power of attraction. Here, one learns to recognize their energetic vibration and how it intertwines with one true love. Through the use of rituals, affirmations, and manifestations, one develops greater awareness and understanding of their thoughts and feelings. This understanding allows individuals to create a greater connection between themselves and the universe, thus increasing their capacity to attract one true love.

The third step focuses on intensifying the connection to the cosmic source of love.

Here, one learns to cultivate a profound understanding of the power of intention and how it can manifest love. Through the use of visualizations and guided meditations, one can access their true inner power and the power of the universe. By consciously connecting to the source of love, one can create the understanding that love is always available to them.

The fourth and final step of the journey involves a deepening of the connection between the individual and their one true love. Here, one acknowledges and accepts the beauty of the love they have attracted and embraces it completely. This step emphasizes the importance of living in the present moment, enjoying each moment fully, and embracing the positive attributes of the relationship.

By following the steps outlined in Manifest the One True Love, individuals can develop a deeper understanding of themselves and the power that lies within. In the end, one is equipped with the knowledge and understanding to create and cultivate a meaningful and lasting relationship. This book is an incredibly valuable guide on self-discovery and creating a life-long love. From the exploration of self-awareness, self-confidence, and self-love to the understanding of the power of attraction, visualizations, and intentional manifestation, this book is an invaluable resource for anyone looking to create and cultivate one true love.

Making the Most of Your Relationship

For those who have taken the time to read the book, Manifest True Love, it is clear that there are simple steps one can take to make the most of their relationship.

The first step is to focus on what brings the two of you joy. People often get stuck in the same old routine, which can quickly become mundane and unfulfilling. To keep the relationship fresh and exciting, it is important to always be exploring new activities you can do together. Making an effort to do something fun and different will open up a whole new world of possibilities.

The second step is to work on communication. It is essential to be able to discuss your feelings and needs openly and honestly to be able to understand and empathize with each other. Working on good communication skills will go a long way toward creating a strong foundation for the relationship.

Thirdly, it is important to make time for each other. It is easy to get caught up in life's responsibilities and forget that time spent together is often the most important factor in fostering and maintaining a relationship. Taking the time to just enjoy each other's company is essential.

Fourthly, it is important to make sure that both parties are putting in equal effort. If one partner is doing more than their fair share, it can create resentment and potential discord.

Making sure that each person takes responsibility for their part in the relationship is essential.

Finally, it is important to understand that relationships take work. Even the most effortless seeming partnerships take hard work and dedication. Making the effort to understand and care for one another will go a long way toward creating a lasting connection.

By following these steps, it is possible to make the most of your relationship and turn it into a strong and lasting bond. Taking time to invest in your relationship and putting in the effort to make it work will result in a lasting connection. Manifest The One True Love is an invaluable resource for couples to use to build the relationship of their dreams.